Published By Adam Gilbin

@ Mike Kong

Wheat Belly Diet Meal Plan: A Gluten-free Path to

Weight Loss and Delicious Dishes Without the

Grain

All Right RESERVED

ISBN 978-87-94477-23-9

TABLE OF CONTENTS

Hot Coconut Flaxseed Cereal 1

Flaxseed Wrap 3

Wheat Free Pancakes 5

Wheatless Bakery 7

Pizza Crust 11

Banana Bread 15

Delectable Blueberry Pancakes 18

Spiced Cranberry Muffins 20

Meatballs With Tomato Sauce 22

Nutty Chicken Nuggets 25

Dairy Free Pancakes 27

Breakfast Bars 28

Orange Plantain 32

Apple Chicken Sausage 35

Carrot Cake 37

Chocolate And Banana Muffins 41

One Skillet Breakfast Scramble 43

- Walnut And Spinach Quiche Cups 45
- Peanut Butter And Chocolate Fudge 47
- Almond And Chocolate Biscotti 49
- Sugar Free Non Bake Cheesecake 52
- Apple Cranberry Crumble 54
- Wheat Free Pumpkin Pie 57
- Baked Eggs With Spinach & Tomato 60
- Fruit Salad With Yogurt 61
- Onion, Garlic & Kale 63
- Quinoa & Black Beans 65
- Perfect Pork Ribs 67
- Vegetable Bake 69
- Cheese Eggplant Bake 71
- Pumpkin Spice Muffins 73
- Garlic Bread 75
- Creamy Yogurt Fresh Fruit Salad 80
- Best Baked Oatmeal 82
- Fiesta Feast Omelets 84

- Back To Basics Skillet Chicken 86
- Ham And Egg Breakfast Meal 88
- Matzo Ball Soup 90
- Silver Dollar Pancakes 92
- Cinnamon Buns 94
- Potatoes With Eggs And Green Beans 97
- Breakfast Smoothies 98
- Blueberry Pancakes 100
- Eggplant And Mango Salad 102
- Chocolate Squares 105
- Coconut And Banana Pie 106
- Baby Spinach And Fennel Salad 109
- Bacon Bleu Cheese Burger Patties 111
- Bacon Lettuce Tomato Salad 113
- Cheddar Broccoli Soup 114
- Bbq Meat Loaf 117
- Chicken With Basil Cream Sauce 119
- Bbq Potatoes 122

Strawberry Banana Smoothie 124

Crusted Chicken Tenders... 125

Glazed Salmon... 127

Vegetable Chili 128

Berry Coconut Smoothie 131

Ginger Blueberry Parfait.. 133

Flourless Honey Almond Cake....................................... 135

Oriental Chicken Salad 137

Chicken Nuggets.. 138

Dreamy Walnut Cake 141

Hot Coconut Flaxseed Cereal

Ingredients:

- ¼ cup unsweetened coconut flakes

- ¼ cup chopped walnuts or raw sunflower seeds

- ¼ cup sliced blueberries, strawberries, or any berries (optional)

- Ground cinnamon

- ½ cup whole dairy milk, coconut milk, unsweetened almond milk, or fullfat soymilk,

- ½ cup ground flaxseeds

Directions::

1. Mix the milk, coconut flakes, and walnuts or sunflower seeds, and ground flaxseeds, in a bowl and put it into the microwave for 1 minute.

2. You can optionally sprinkle with cinnamon and some berries before serving.

Flaxseed Wrap

Ingredients:

- ¼ teaspoon paprika
- 1 tablespoon water
- 1 tablespoon coconut oil
- 1 large egg
- 3 tablespoons ground flaxseeds
- ¼ teaspoon onion powder
- ¼ teaspoon baking powder
- Sea salt

Directions::

1. Put the ground baking powder, flaxseeds, paprika, onion powder, and seas salt together in a bowl.

2. Mix in a tablespoon coconut oil. Crack in an egg and 1 tablespoon water, mix well.
3. Grease a microwavable pie pan using coconut oil. Put in the batter and spread consistently at the bottom.
4. Microwave it on high level for at least 2 up to 3 minutes until it is cooked. Let it sit for about 5 minutes to cool down.
5. In order to remove it, lift up the edges using the spatula. You can use pancake turner to mildly loosen from the pan if it sticks.

Wheat Free Pancakes

Ingredients:

- ½ teaspoon of sea salt

- ½ teaspoon of baking soda

- ¾ cup unsweetened almond milk (milk or light coconut milk can serve as a good replacement)

- 3 cups of almond meal

- 1 tablespoon of ground flaxseeds

- 2 tablespoons extralight olive oil (can be replaced with walnut oil, butter or coconut oil)

Directions::

1. The almond meal, salt, flaxseeds and baking soda are mixed in a medium bowl
2. Whisk the eggs in a large bowl

3. Add milk and oil into the eggs and whisk
4. Progressively add the flour mixture into the egg mixture as you whisk
5. Whisk until you get a consistent batter
6. Heat a large skillet over medium heat
7. Lightly add oil to the skillet
8. Pour ¼ cup of the batter onto the griddle and cook for 3 minutes
9. Turn and cook for another 3 minutes
10. Repeat the process until all batter is finished

Wheatless Bakery

Ingredients:

To make flavored oil you will need:

- 12 tablespoons of minced basil or rosemary
- 2 large cloves garlic minced
- 3 tablespoons of olive oil
- ½ teaspoon of fine sea salt

To make the dough you will need:

- ½ teaspoon fine sea salt
- 1 teaspoon of rapid rise yeast (optional)
- 1cup buttermilk
- 4egg whites
- 2 cups almond meal or flour
- 2 tablespoons of baking powder

- 1cup garbanzo bean flour

- ½ cup ground golden flaxseeds

Directions::

To make flavored oil:

1. Place a small saucepan over low heat
2. Put in the salt oil and garlic
3. Simmer for 10 minutes
4. If using rosemary add it and simmer for another 10 minutes
5. Remove saucepan from heat
6. If using basil add it to the oil
7. At this stage preheat the oven to 400o F
8. Take 13 by 9inch baking sheet and grease it with half of the oil
9. Line it with parchment paper
10. Brush the paper with the remaining oil

To make dough:

11. Combine the almond meal or flour, flaxseeds, baking powder, salt and garbanzo bean flour in a large bowl.
12. Whisk until well broken up and properly mixed
13. Add yeast and buttermilk into a small bowl and whisk until the yeast dissolves
14. Beat the eggs in another bowl until stiff peaks form
15. Mix the yeast and the flour mixture until it forms rough dough balls
16. Gently fold in the egg whites till they are fairly well incorporated
17. Using a spatula spread the dough in the pan
18. Use your fingertips to dimple the top of the dough
19. Pour remaining oil mixture on the dough and cover them entirely with the oil.
20. Bake for about 20minutesuntil golden brown and slightly spongy in the center

21. Cut into desired size using a knife or pizza bread.

Pizza Crust

Ingredients:

- ¾ teaspoon of salt
- 1 teaspoon of thickener
- 1cup warm water
- 1 ½ teaspoons of moment yeast
- 2 tablespoons of olive oil for the batter
- 2 tablespoons of olive oil for the pan
- 1 ½ cups of earthy colored rice flour
- 2 tablespoons nonfat milk powder (dry) or buttermilk powder
- 1 teaspoon of baking powder
- 1tablespoon honey or sugar

Directions::

1. Preheat the stove to 425 degrees Fahrenheit.
2. Put the dry fixings in general, with the exception of the yeast, in a huge blending bowl. The stand blender's bowl is ideal for this. Blend everything until completely incorporated.
3. In a little bowl, include the olive oil, warm water, yeast, and about portion of the dry combination. Mix until everything is consolidated. Assuming there are still a few protuberances, that is okay.
4. Leave the combination for around 30 minutes. You will see that the blend turns out to be effervescent and will begin to have a yeasty smell.
5. Add the past combination to the excess dry fixings. Beat everything on medium high velocity for around 4 minutes.
6. The subsequent combination will be tacky and thick. It is ideal to utilize a stand or electric

hand blender to ensure everything is very much fused. Hand blending is not exactly right enough.

7. Let the mixture rest while covered for around 30 minutes or so.
8. Drizzle the 2 tablespoons of olive oil onto a baking sheet or a 12" width pizza container. Take out the batter from the bowl and on the oil puddle.
9. With wet fingers, begin working the mixture outwards beginning at the middle. Press it into a 12to 14inch circle.
10. Let the batter rest again for 15 minutes, this time without a cover.
11. Bake it for around 810 minutes or until everything is set. You will know it when the surface beginnings looking misty rather than shiny.
12. Remove this from the broiler and afterward top it with anything that you need.

13. Return everything to the broiler for around 1015 minutes, or relying upon the garnishes that you have chosen.
14. Serve warm.

Banana Bread

Ingredients:

- 1 cup of sugar
- 1/3 cup of sunflower oil
- ½ cup of unsweetened fruit purée
- 1 teaspoon of vanilla extract
- ½ cup slashed pecans
- 2 cups of corn flour
- 1 teaspoon of baking soft drink
- 4 eggs
- ¼ teaspoon of salt
- 2 cups of ready bananas, squashed (around 45 medium bananas)

Directions::

1. Preheat the broiler to 350° Fahrenheit.
2. In a major bowl, blend the salt, corn flour, and baking pop. Ensure that everything is blended well.
3. In a little bowl, whisk the sugar, eggs, oil, bananas, and vanilla. Ensure that everything is well incorporated.
4. Add the wet combination to the dry fixings and mix until the dry Ingredients: are moistened.
5. Coat the surfaces of 2 8x4inch portion dish with cooking shower.
6. Sprinkle the base with the hacked walnuts. Empty the blend into the two portion pans.
7. Bake the bread for around 4555 minutes. You can check assuming it's now cooked through the toothpick test (embed a toothpick close to the focal point of the bread and it should come out clean).

8. Cool the bread for around 10 minutes or so before you take them out from the portion skillet and onto wire racks.
9. This bread is amazing along with tea or espresso. For the people who wish to have a cool treat for warm days, this bread likewise functions admirably when left in the cooler to cool.

Delectable Blueberry Pancakes

Ingredients:

- 1/2 tablespoon vegetable oil
- 1 teaspoon vanilla
- 1/2 cup fresh blueberries
- Syrup of your choice
- 1 cup rice flour
- 1/2 tablespoon sugar
- 1 teaspoon baking
- 1 pinch of salt
- 1/4 cup skim milk
- 1 small egg

Directions::

1. Heat a greased skillet on medium high heat on the stove.
2. As the skillet heats, mix all the wet Ingredients: in a large mixing bowl, then all the dry Ingredients: in another mixing bowl.
3. Combine all the wet and dry Ingredients: in the larger bowl, and then add the blueberries.
4. Use a ladle and divide the batter into even portions on the skillet.
5. Cook until golden brown, about three minutes on each side. Serve with the syrup of your choice.
6. Wheat free and delicious, these pancakes are the perfect way to start your healthy eating for the day!

Spiced Cranberry Muffins

Ingredients:

- 1 small egg
- 1/2 cup coconut milk
- 1 tablespoon vegetable oil
- ½ cup cranberry raisins
- 1 teaspoon cinnamon
- 1 cup potato flour
- 1/4 cup sugar
- 1 teaspoon baking powder
- 1 pinch of salt

Directions::

1. Preheat your oven to 400 degrees F, and line six muffin cups with paper.

2. Mix all of the dry Ingredients: together, making a hole in the middle of the mixture in the bowl.
3. In a separate dish, combine all of the wet Ingredients:, and then add to the dry Ingredients:. Mix until everything is just combined, then add in the cranberries.
4. Pour batter into the muffin cups, and bake at 400 degrees F for 20 minutes. Let cool before serving or storing.
5. A perfect and delicious way to start your day, these wheat free muffins are so delicious, you won't believe how healthy they really are!

Meatballs With Tomato Sauce

Ingredients:

- ¼ cup Parmesan cheese
- 2 lightly beaten eggs
- 1/3 cup whole wheat bread crumbs
- 12 oz. or 3 pieces sausages removed from casings
- 1 lb. ground beef (choose one with less fat)
- 1 tsp. minced garlic
- Salt
- Pepper
- Parmesan cheese for garnish

Sauce:

- 1 tbsp. Minced garlic

- 2 cans tomatoes, diced and pureed
- 1 tsp. Dried oregano
- 2 tsp. Dried basil
- Salt

Directions::

1. Preheat the oven to 425° F. Remove the sausages and ground beef from the cold.
2. Squeeze the sausage meat from their casings and bring both meats to room temperature.
3. Put the bread crumbs in a bowl and add 1/3 cup of hot water. Let the crumbs absorb the water before adding the garlic, salt, pepper, grated Parmesan cheese and the eggs.
4. After mixing them well, add the meats and use your hands to combine them.
5. Prepare the pan or dish with oil or nonstick spray. Round up meatballs with your hands, using a spoon to measure out the meat.

Arrange them so they'll have space between each meatball.
6. Puree the tomatoes. After putting it in a bowl, add in the salt, herbs and garlic. Pour this sauce over the meatballs. Sprinkle the remaining cheese over them. Bake them until the sauce and the cheese is bubbling. That would take just over half an hour.
7. Serve it hot with more Parmesan sprinkled on the meatballs.

Nutty Chicken Nuggets

Ingredients:

- ½ cup almond flour or almond meal
- ½ tsp. chicken seasoning
- 2 skinless chicken breasts, boneless
- 2 tbsp. olive oil
- 1 tsp. paprika

Directions::

1. Preheat oven to 400° F. Prepare the pan and baking sheet with the olive oil.
2. Remove all tendons and visible fat from the chicken then cut it into nuggets (each breast piece should make about 5 pieces). Make sure they are all of the same thickness, using a kitchen mallet to even out differences.

3. Combine the rest of the Ingredients: in a bowl and mix well. Dip each nugget into this mixture, making sure it coats the chicken evenly. Line them up into the pan with the baking sheet.
4. Cook for around 10 minutes, until the side touching the pan is slightly browned. The nuggets become too hard and chewy when overcooked so don't overdo it.
5. Once one side is cooked, turn the nuggets and then cook for another 10 minutes.
6. Serve hot with your favorite chicken nugget dip.

Dairy Free Pancakes

Ingredients:

- ½ tsp of cinnamon
- 3 pcs of large eggs
- 5 tbsp of full fat coconut milk
- 2 tbsp of honey
- 1 tsp of vanilla
- ¼ cup of strawberries
- 1 ½ cups of finely ground blanched almond flour
- ½ tsp of baking soda
- ¼ tsp of salt
- Oil, for cooking

Directions::

1. Prepare a large mixing bowl. Sift the almond flour, baking soda, salt, and cinnamon into the bowl and stir to combine.
2. In a separate mixing bowl, add in the eggs, coconut milk, honey, and vanilla. Whisk the Ingredients: together until properly incorporated. Pour the mixture into the mixing bowl with the flour mixture.
3. Stir the Ingredients: until they form a smooth batter. Then, set the mixture aside.
4. Prepare a skillet and heat the oil. Don't let the pan get too hot or the pancakes will stick.
5. Pour the batter into the pan and lower the heat if necessary.
6. Flip the pancake once the edges are just starting to form and the topside is bubbly. Fry until the pancake is cooked through. Top with honey or maple syrup and sliced fruits.

Breakfast Bars

Ingredients:

- ½ cup of unsweetened shredded coconut
- ½ cup of pumpkin seeds
- ½ cup of sunflower seeds
- ¼ cup of blanched slivered almonds
- ¼ cup of raisins
- 1 ¼ cup of almond flour (pick the blanched variant)
- ¼ tsp of bay salt (rock salt should be fine)
- ¼ tsp of baking soda
- ¼ cup of grape seed oil
- ¼ cup of agave nectar
- 1 tsp of vanilla extract

Directions::

1. In a small mixing bowl, combine the almond flour, baking soda, and Celtic sea salt. Stir the Ingredients: together.
2. In a large mixing bowl, combine the grapeseed oil, vanilla extract, and agave nectar. Stir until the Ingredients: are well mixed. Gradually add in the almond flour mixture into the bowl and mix well.
3. Add in the shredded coconut, pumpkin seeds, almond slivers, sunflower seeds, and raisins. Stir the Ingredients: together until well incorporated.
4. Prepare an 8" x 8" baking dish and slightly grease it using the grapeseed oil. Place the dough on the baking dish. Spread it evenly and pat it down using a spatula or with your bare hands.
5. Place the baking dish inside the oven and bake for 20 minutes at 350°F. Once cooking time is done, place the bars on a cooling pan

and let them cool for two hours before serving.

Orange Plantain

Ingredients:

- ¾ c. Polenta, instant
- ¼ c. Greek yogurt
- ¼ c. Mascarpone
- 1 tsp. Chopped tarragon
- 4 tbsp. Honey
- 1 orange
- 2 c. Water
- ¼ tsp. Salt
- 1 ½ c. Milk

Directions::

1. To start this recipe, you will want to zest your orange so that you end up with about 1 ½ teaspoons. Set this zest aside for now.
2. Take the rest of the orange peel and get rid of the white pith and cut off the segments before setting this aside to use as the garnish.
3. Next, take the salt, water, and milk and combine them in a saucepan on the stove. Bring the mixture to boil while slowly whisking in the polenta and letting it all come to a boil. You will then want to reduce the heat of the mixture and let the polenta have time to thicken, which will take about 5 minutes.
4. After that time, take everything from the heat, cover it up, and give it 5 more minutes to stand and set.
5. While the polenta is setting, you can bring out a bowl and combined ½ teaspoon orange zest, 1 tablespoon honey, yogurt, and mascarpone together.

6. When the plantain is done, you can add in the rest of the orange zest and the honey.
7. Divide this between 4 bowls before topping with a little bit of the mascarpone.
8. Garnish with the orange segments and some tarragon before serving this dish right away.

Apple Chicken Sausage

Ingredients:

- 1 Tbsp. packed brown sugar
- ¾ tsp. salt
- ½ tsp. fennel seed
- ¼ tsp. ground pepper
- 1diced onion
- 2 tsp. canola oil
- 1 apple
- 1 Tbsp. chopped sage
- 1 lb. chicken

Directions::

1. To start this recipe, you should heat up the oil on a skillet before adding in the onion. Allow

the onion to cook for around 2 minutes so that it starts to soften.
2. Add the apples n next and let it cook for another 2 minutes. After this time, move the two Ingredients: to a bowl and let them cool for about 5 minutes.
3. Take the pepper, salt, fennel, sugar, sage, and chicken and add them into the bowl as well and mix gently to combine.
4. Using the same pan as before, place 4 portions of this mixture back into the pan, making sure to flatten them so that they become patties. Cook these patties so they become fully cooked through, which will take about 3 minutes on each side.
5. Repeat these steps until all of the mixture is gone and then enjoy!

Carrot Cake

Ingredients:

- Vanilla 1 teaspoon
- Apple cider vinegar 1 teaspoon
- Coconut flour 2 cups
- Cinnamon 1 teaspoon
- Baking soda 2 teaspoon
- Coconut 1 cup (shredded)
- Nuts 1 cup (chopped)
- Water 1 cup
- Eggs 4 large
- Carrots 2 cups (grated)
- Honey ¼ cup
- Raisins ½ cup

- Flax meal 2 tablespoon

- Sugar 1 cup

- Olive oil 0 1 ¼ cup

- Salt 1 teaspoon

Directions::

1. In a small sauce pan put raisins and water and bring to a boil; then reduce heat, cover and simmer until raisins are soft and swollen.
2. Take a small bowl and mix flax meal and water together and stand for a couple of minutes before mixing into batter.
3. In a medium sized bowl beat sugar and eggs until smooth and add flax meal and water mixture and combine well.
4. Add oil, honey, and vanilla and mix until well combined.
5. Add raisins and apple cider vinegar to the mixture and stir well.
6. Add the coconut flour, cinnamon, salt and baking soda and mix well.
7. Add grated carrots, coconut and nuts and blend well.
8. Pour the mass into the prepared and greased pan and spread.

9. Bake for 50–60 minutes at 200°c

Chocolate And Banana Muffins

Ingredients:

- Chocolate chips ¼ cup
- Baking soda ¼ teaspoon
- Olive oil ¼ cup
- Honey ¼ cup
- Salt ¼ teaspoon
- Bananas 3 ripe (mashed)
- Eggs 3
- Coconut flour 3 tablespoons
- Cocoa powder 1/3 cup

Directions::

1. Take a medium sized bowl and combine all Ingredients: except for the chocolate chips; mix until well combined.
2. Take a muffin tins and line with liners; fill with batter for about 2/3 and top with chocolate chips.
3. Insert into the preheated oven of 200°c and bake for 15 to 20 minutes.

One Skillet Breakfast Scramble

Ingredients:

- Cumin: 1/4 teaspoon

- Eggs: 4 large

- Garlic: 1 tablespoon, Minced

- Green Onion: ½ cup, chopped

- Olive Oil: 1 tablespoon plus 1 teaspoon

- Baby spinach: 2 cups, chopped

- Black Pepper: 1/2 teaspoon

- Breakfast Sausage: ½ pound, crumbled

Directions::

1. Heat one tablespoon of olive oil, green onion and minced garlic in a large skillet over medium heat until onion softens, about 5 minutes.

2. Add sausage crumbles and cook, stirring frequently until just sausage is cooked, about 67 minutes.
3. While sausage is cooking crack eggs into a bowl and add remaining olive oil, pepper, and cumin, scramble with whisk.
4. Pour eggs into skillet with sausage, onions and garlic, stir frequently until eggs start to set.
5. Add spinach and continue cooking, stirring constantly until eggs are done, about 5 minutes.

Walnut And Spinach Quiche Cups

Ingredients:

- Sea Salt: 1/2 teaspoon

- Turmeric: 1/2 teaspoon

- Walnuts: ½ cup, chopped

- Baby spinach: 2 cups, chopped

- Cinnamon: 1/4 teaspoon

- Eggs: 6 large

- Milk: 2 tablespoons

Directions::

1. Heat oven to 350°.
2. Combine eggs and milk in a glass bowl, mix until smooth, add other Ingredients: and mix well.

3. Coat the cups of a 12slot muffin pan with nonstick spray. Spoon egg mixture into the muffin cups until each is about 1/2 full.
4. Place in oven and cook until done, about 20 minutes.

Peanut Butter And Chocolate Fudge

Ingredients:

- 8 ounces chocolate, unsweetened
- 1 tsp. vanilla
- 4 ounces lowfat cream cheese, melted
- ½ cup walnuts, chopped
- Coconut oil, melted
- 1 cup peanut butter, smooth
- Sea salt

Directions::

1. Lightly grease the bottom of an 8x8inch baking pan with the melted coconut oil. Set the pan to the side for the moment.

2. Place the melted cream cheese, peanut butter and vanilla extract in a bowl. Stir until well combined. Set to the side for the moment.
3. Melt the chocolate in the microwave using a microwavesafe bowl at 30second intervals, stirring after each interval, until the chocolate has melted completely.
4. Slowly add the chocolate to the cream cheese mixture, stirring until well combined. Fold in the chopped walnuts.
5. Spread the fudge into the prepared baking pan from Step 1. Set the fudge to the side and let set. Once it has harden a bit, cut the fudge into squares.

Almond And Chocolate Biscotti

Ingredients:

- 2 large eggs
- ½ cup ricotta cheese
- ¼ cup cocoa powder, unsweetened
- 1 tsp. almond extract
- 2 ½ ounces dark chocolate, chopped
- ½ cup slivered almonds, toasted
- ¼ cup coconut oil, melted
- ¼ cup xylitol
- ¼ cup almond butter, softened
- ¼ cup almond milk, unsweetened
- 2 Tbsp. coconut flour

- 3 cups almond flour

Directions::

1. Turn the oven on to 350degrees and let preheat. Prepare a baking sheet by lining it with parchment paper. Set to the side.
2. In a mixing bowl, whisk together all the eggs, xylitol, milk, coconut oil, almond extract and ricotta cheese together.
3. Stir in the remaining Ingredients:. Continue to mix until smooth.
4. Using your hands, shape the mixture into a loaflike shape and set it on the baking sheet from Step 1.
5. Place the baking sheet in the oven and bake for about 40 to 45 minutes.
6. Remove the biscotti from the oven and let cool. Turn the oven down to 300degrees.
7. Cut the load into slices about 3inches thick. Place the biscotti back in the oven and bake

for an additional 30 to 35 minutes, making sure to term them over while baking.

Sugar Free Non Bake Cheesecake

Ingredients:

- 2 packages cheesecake pudding, sugarfree and fatfree
- 2 cups fruit, such as blueberries or strawberries
- 1 graham cracker pie shell, lowfat
- 1 container whip cream, fatfree
- 2 cups milk, nonfat

Directions::

1. Open both packages of the pudding and dump them into a bowl. Add the milk and stir until well dissolved.
2. Evenly spread about half of the pudding mixture into the graham cracker pie shell.

3. Sprinkle 1 cup of the fruit on top of the pudding mixture. Use your fingers to gently press the fruit into the pudding.
4. Stir half of the whip cream into the remaining pudding mixture. Spread this mixture overtop the fruit.
5. Spread the other half of the whip cream on top, followed by the remaining cup of fruit.
6. Place the cheesecake in the fridge and let set for about 2 hours.

Apple Cranberry Crumble

Ingredients:

Crust and crumble topping

- 1½ teaspoons ground cinnamon
- 1 tablespoon molasses
- 1½ teaspoons vanilla extract
- 3 cups almond meal
- 1 stick (8 tablespoons) butter, softened
- 1 cup xylitol (or other sweetener equivalent to 1 cup sugar)
- Dash sea salt

Filling

- 1 Granny Smith apple (or other variety)
- 1 teaspoon ground cinnamon

- 1 cup fresh cranberries

- 16 ounces cream cheese, softened

- 2 large eggs

- ½ cup xylitol (or other sweetener equivalent to ½ cup sugar)

Directions:

1. Preheat oven to 350° F. In large bowl, combine almond meal, butter, sweetener, cinnamon, molasses, vanilla, and salt and mix.
2. Grease a 9½inch tart or pie pan. Using approximately 1 cup of the almond meal mixture, form a thin bottom crust with your hands or spoon.
3. In another bowl, combine cream cheese, eggs, and sweetener and mix with spoon or mixer at low speed. Pour into tart or pie pan.
4. Core apple and slice into very thin sections.

5. Arrange in circles around the edge of the cream cheese mixture, working inwards. Distribute cranberries over top, then sprinkle cinnamon over entire mixture.
6. Gently layer remaining almond meal crumble evenly over top. Bake for 30 minutes or until topping lightly browned.

Wheat Free Pumpkin Pie

Ingredients:

Pie crust

- 1 teaspoon ground cinnamon
- 1 teaspoon unsweetened cocoa powder
- 1 large egg
- 4 ounces butter or coconut oil, melted
- 1 1/4 cups ground walnuts (or pecans or almonds)
- 1/4 cup ground flaxseed

Pie filling

- 2 teaspoons ground cinnamon
- 1 1/2 teaspoons ground nutmeg

- 1 teaspoon ground ginger
- Sweetener equivalent to 1 cup sugar (e.g., 6 tablespoons Truvia)
- 2 cups pumpkin puree
- 8 ounces cream cheese, softened
- 2 large eggs
- 1/2 cup coconut milk (canned variety)
- 2 teaspoons vanilla extract

Directions:

1. Preheat oven to 350 degrees F. In large bowl, mix together ground walnuts, flaxseed, cinnamon, and cocoa powder. In small bowl, whisk eggs and add butter or coconut oil. Pour liquid mix into dry mix and blend by hand thoroughly.
2. Grease a 9inch pie pan with coconut oil or other oil. Transfer mix to the pie pan and

spread evenly along bottom and up sides. If mixture is too thin, place in refrigerator for several minutes to thicken.
3. For ease of spreading, use a large metal spoon heated under running hot water. Set aside.
4. In another large bowl, combine pumpkin, cream cheese, eggs, coconut milk, and vanilla extract and mix thoroughly by hand.
5. Add cinnamon, nutmeg, ginger, and sweetener and continue to blend by hand.
6. Pour pumpkin mix into pie crust. Bake in oven for 40 minutes or until toothpick or knife withdraws nearly dry.
7. Optionally, sprinkle additional nutmeg and/or cinnamon, top with whipped cream or whipped coconut milk.

Baked Eggs With Spinach & Tomato

Ingredients:

- ½ cup bag spinach

- 1 cup chopped tomatoes

- ½ teaspoon chilli flakes

- 2 eggs

Directions:

1. Heat the Oven to 300° F.
2. Wash spinach leaves with boiling water. Drain and divide in 2 small oven safe plates.
3. Mix tomatoes with chili flakes and a little spice, then add mixture to spinach. Make a small hole in the center of each and break an egg.
4. Bake for 1215 minutes. Serve with crusty bread, if desired.

Fruit Salad With Yogurt

Ingredients:

Fruits:

- 1 small honeydew melon
- 1 pint strawberries
- ¼ tbsp. fresh lime juice
- 1 small watermelon
- 1 tablespoon honey

Lime yogurt:

- 1 cups nonfat plain yogurt
- ¼ cup sugar

Directions:

1. Cut watermelon and honeydew melon to small bite sized pieces

2. In a large bowl, mix watermelon, melon, strawberries, lime juice and honey.
3. In a separate small bowl, mix yogurt, sugar.
4. When ready layer the fruits and yogurt and enjoy.

Onion, Garlic & Kale

Ingredients:

- 3 tbsp olive oil

- 1 onion, chopped

- 3 bunches kale washed, dried, and shredded

- 3 cloves garlic, minced

- 1 cup bread crumbs

Directions:

1. Warm 1tbsp of olive oil over high heat in a nonstick skillet.
2. Toss in the garlic and onion. Cook for 57 minutes or until both the garlic and onion have softened.
3. Toss in the breadcrumbs and mix to incorporate. Cook for 23 minutes or until the breadcrumbs have browned.

4. Throw in the kale and cook for another 23 minutes, or until the kale has wilted. Stir throughout to ensure the vegetables do not burn.

Quinoa & Black Beans

Ingredients:

- 1 tbsp sunflower oil
- 1 onion, chopped
- 4 cloves garlic, chopped
- ½ tsp cayenne pepper
- A pinch of salt & pepper
- 1 cup frozen corn kernels
- 14oz canned black beans, rinsed and drained
- 1 ½ cups vegetable broth
- 1 tsp ground cumin
- 1 cup quinoa

Directions:

1. In a medium saucepan, warm 1 tbsp sunflower oil. Toss in the garlic and onion and cook for 57 minutes or until both vegetables have softened.
2. Combine quinoa with the onion and garlic, stirring to ensure an even distribution. Add the vegetable broth and throw in all the seasonings except the cilantro.
3. Cover the saucepan and lower the heat until a gentle simmer is produced. Cook for 20 minutes.
4. Toss in the corn and cook for 5 minutes. Finally, throw in the cilantro and the black beans.
5. Heat for a moment or two to ensure the beans are warm. Serve immediately.

Perfect Pork Ribs

Ingredients:

- 2 bay leaves
- 1 teaspoon of coriander seed
- 1 teaspoon of mustard seed
- 1 teaspoon of peppercorn
- 1 ½ kg of pork ribs
- 350g of barbecue sauce
- 2 pork stock cubes

Directions:

1. Place four tablespoons of your chosen barbecue sauce in your slow cooker with all the other Ingredients:.

2. Add extra water to ensure that the pork ribs are submerged in liquid. Slow cook for around 8 hours and 30 minutes.
3. 30 minutes before serving, preheat your oven to 425F or gas mark 7.
4. Remove the ribs from the slow cooker gently; the meat will be incredibly soft and may break apart if handled without finesse.
5. Coat the ribs using the leftover barbecue sauce.
6. Place on a baking tray and cover with tin foil. Cook for 25 minutes or until the rib skin has become crisp. Serve when ready.

Vegetable Bake

Ingredients:

- Chili flakes
- 300g eggplant
- 2 zucchinis
- ½ jar of roasted red peppers
- 3 beefsteak tomatoes
- Torn basil
- 4 garlic cloves
- 400g chopped tomatoes
- Oregano
- 250g mozzarella balls

Directions:

1. Place your slow onto a high setting.

2. Crush three garlic cloves and add these to your slow cooker alongside the chopped tomatoes, a pinch of chili flakes, oregano and salt.
3. Cover these Ingredients: and leave to slow cook for several moments.
4. Chop the eggplant, zucchini, red peppers and beefsteak tomatoes into moderate sized slices.
5. Remove the tomato sauce from the slow cooker. Take your vegetable slices and place half of them in layers in your slow cooker.
6. Cover these layers in half your tomato sauce, a pinch of chili, oregano and half your mozzarella.
7. Repeat once more for the remaining Ingredients:. Cover and slow cook for 6 hours and 30 minutes. Serve with salad or a side of your choice.

Cheese Eggplant Bake

Ingredients:

- 1 cup shredded whole milk mozzarella cheese
- 2 tomatoes
- 2 cups tomato sauce
- 3 minced cloves garlic
- 4 tablespoons sundried tomatoes
- 5 chopped fresh basil leaves
- ½ cup virgin olive oil
- ½ cup grated Parmesan cheese
- 1 cup ricotta cheese
- 1 cut crosswise eggplant
- 1 chopped onion
- 6 cups spinach leaves

Directions:

1. Preheat your oven to 175°C. Put the slices of eggplant in the baking pan.
2. Cover both sides of slices with oil. Bake it for 15 to 20 minutes.
3. Take out the eggplant out but leave your oven on. Heat the 2 tablespoons of oil in a skillet in medium heat.
4. Put in the garlic, onion, spinach, and sundried tomatoes, and cook it until the onion softens.
5. Toss the tomato over the eggplant. Lay the spinach mix over it. Put in the tomato sauce over the spinach.
6. Add in the mozzarella and ricotta cheeses in the bowl. Spread in the two types of cheese on the tomato sauce and put the basil over.
7. Add in the Parmesan cheese over it. Bake for about 30 minutes without any cover. You will know it is ready when the cheese starts to melt.

Pumpkin Spice Muffins

Ingredients:

- 1 teaspoon ground allspice
- 1 teaspoon grated nutmeg
- 1 teaspoon baking powder
- 2 cups ground almonds
- 2 teaspoons ground cinnamon
- 1 can unsweetened pumpkin puree
- Fine sea salt
- Sweetener like stevia extract, Truvia, or Splenda
- ¼ cup ground flaxseeds
- ¼ cup melted coconut oil, walnut oil, or olive oil

- ½ cup sour cream or coconut milk
- 1 cup chopped walnuts
- 2 large eggs

Directions:

1. Preheat your oven to 175°C. Grease up about 12 cup muffin tin using oil.
2. Mix together the walnuts, almond meal, sweetener, ground flaxseeds, allspice, cinnamon, baking powder, nutmeg, and salt in a bowl.
3. Mix together the sour cream or coconut milk, pumpkin, oil, and eggs in another bowl.
4. Mix the pumpkin mixture and almond meal mixture together carefully.
5. Put batter into the cup muffin tins. Bake in the oven for about 45 minutes. Cool down and serve.

Garlic Bread

Ingredients:

Wet

- 1/3 cup of entire psyllium husks
- 1/3 cup of ground chia seeds
- 2 ½ cups of warm water (around 105110°F)
- 1 teaspoon honey
- 2 tablespoons maple syrup
- 2 ¼ teaspoons of dynamic dry yeast
- 2 tablespoons of additional virgin olive oil (in addition to extra for topping)

Dry

- 1 cup sorghum flour
- ½ cup sweet rice flour

- 1 cup teff flour

- ½ cup almond meal

- 1 ½ teaspoons of ocean salt

Directions:

1. When you purchase entire chia seeds, utilize an espresso processor to crush them. Store the ground chia seeds in a glass container and pop it in the cooler just until a week.
2. Preheat the stove to 400° Fahrenheit.
3. Put the warm water in a bowl. Consolidate a teaspoon of honey and the yeast and whisk them together.
4. Leave the blend for around 510 minutes to allow the yeast to actuate. The combination ought to turn out to be effervescent or frothy. In the event that this doesn't occur, dispose of the combination and start over.
5. While the yeast is being actuated, you can begin blending the dry fixings in a major bowl.

6. When the yeast is enacted, include the maple syrup, olive oil, psyllium husks, and ground chia seeds into the blend. Leave the blend for around 23 minutes (this is significant, so watch an opportunity) to let the psyllium and the chia seeds discharge a gelatin like substance. Whisk these together.
7. Pour every one of the wet fixings into the bowl with the dry fixings. Combine everything as one utilizing a wooden spoon until the combination turns out to be thick. On a floured wooden board, manipulate the batter to blend in the flour.
8. Add the newly slashed garlic as you work. Add a greater amount of the sorghum and teff flours, a little at a time. Keep adding until the mixture keeps yet is still a piece tacky to the touch.

9. Make a ball with the batter and set it back into the enormous bowl. Cover it with a clammy towel.
10. Place the bowl in a warm spot with the goal that the batter rises. Some put the bowl on a pot that has warm water. Allow it to ascend until the batter is multiplied in size.
11. When the mixture has risen, put a pizza stone inside the broiler. Set a container of water on the base rack, just underneath the pizza stone. You can utilize a 8x8inch glass container loaded up with water (about ¾ of the way).
12. Punch the mixture down and spread it out onto a wooden board that has been gently floured. Ply it for about a moment and afterward structure it into a ball.
13. Put the mixture on a square piece of material paper. Utilizing a sharp blade, make a shallow example on top (a spasm tactoe design).

Shower the top with olive oil, and afterward sprinkle with sesame and poppy seeds. Allow the mixture to ascend for 30 minutes more in a warm place.

14. Carefully lift the material paper with the batter, and put it on the stone inside the stove. Prepare the bread for 40 minutes.
15. Remove the bread from the stove once cooked, and let it cool for around 30an hour prior to cutting it. The bread is still a piece sticky in surface when hot and recently out of the oven.

Creamy Yogurt Fresh Fruit Salad

Ingredients:

- 1 8ounce compartment of vanilla or plain yogurt
- 1 teaspoon sugar
- 2 teaspoons lemon juice
- ½ teaspoon vanilla extract
- Lime juice
- 2 cups strawberries, sliced
- 2 bananas, sliced
- 2 new peaches, sliced
- 2 cups grapes

Directions:

1. Mix all the natural product together in a major bowl
2. Mix in around 3 tablespoons of lime juice to keep the natural products from going brown. This likewise assists with supporting the flavor.
3. Mix yogurt, sugar, lemon juice, and vanilla in a little bowl.
4. You have the choice to either serve the yogurt blend as a plunge for the organic products, or blend it right in with the natural product to make a salad.
5. Serve right away

Best Baked Oatmeal

Ingredients:

- 3/4 cup skim milk //
- Pinch of salt
- 1/4 cup raisins
- 1 teaspoon cinnamon
- 1 cup rolled oats
- 2 tablespoons honey
- 3 tablespoons peanut butter

Directions:

1. Preheat your oven to 350 degrees F, and then mix all of the Ingredients: except for the peanut butter in a mixing bowl.

2. Grease a small baking dish with no stick spray, and add the oatmeal mixture to the dish. Bake in the oven for 25 minutes.
3. Melt the peanut butter on the stove or in the microwave and drizzle over the top.
4. A breakfast so tasty it feels like dessert!

Fiesta Feast Omelets

Ingredients:

- 1 corn tortilla
- 1/4 cup light sour cream
- 1/4 cup shredded cheese
- 2 eggs
- 1/4 cup skim milk
- 1/4 chopped green pepper
- 1/4 cup salsa
- 1 small chopped onion

Directions:

1. Scramble the eggs and milk together in a medium saucepan, add in the pepper, onion, and half the sour cream.

2. Spread the remaining sour cream on the tortilla, and pour the eggs in the middle. Add the salsa and cheese on top, then wrap into a burrito. Serve immediately.
3. Some people are surprised at all the ways they can have bread products and avoid wheat, and tortillas are no exception.
4. Use a corn tortilla, and you will have nothing to worry about.
5. A filling fiesta for your mouth, this low calorie and tasty breakfast will keep you full and burning calories all morning long!

Back To Basics Skillet Chicken

Ingredients:

- 1 chopped onion
- 4 crushed garlic cloves
- 1 ½ lbs. boneless chicken
- 3 tbsp. olive oil
- ½ chopped green pepper
- Salt
- Pepper

Directions:

1. Slice the chicken to your desired serving pieces.
2. Heat the oil in the skillet and cook the chicken until they are nearly done.

3. Add the garlic, onion and the green pepper, sauté them with the chicken.
4. You know you are finished cooking when the chicken is slightly browned and the onion has become soft.
5. After that, you can add some choice vegetables and sauté until cooked to your liking.
6. Season with salt and pepper.

Ham And Egg Breakfast Meal

Ingredients:

- 4 large eggs

- 8 slices of black forest ham

- Salt and ground pepper (salt is recommended to be coarse)

- Fresh chives, chopped into bits

Directions:

1. Preheat oven to 350° F. Prepare the pan and baking sheet with the olive oil.
2. Place four pieces of the ham on the baking pan and fold them in such a way that they have a "basket," folding the edges towards the center.
3. Crack an egg on each of the "basket" (you can use a muffin pan to make your life easier with

the hams), and cover with bits of the remaining ham.
4. Season with salt and pepper, then bake until the egg white has set, but with the yolk still runny. That would take about 12 minutes.
5. Top with the chopped chives and serve hot.

Matzo Ball Soup

Ingredients:

- ¼ tsp of pepper

- 2 cups of blanched almond flour, already sifted

- 6 cups of chicken or vegetable stock

- 4 pcs of eggs

- 2 tsp of Celtic sea salt

Directions:

1. In a mixing bowl, add in the eggs, pepper, and 1 teaspoon of salt. Beat the Ingredients: together for 2 minutes.
2. Add in the almond flour and stir. Place the bowl inside the refrigerator and wait for 4 hours.

3. Place a large pot on a stove and fill it with water. Add in the remaining teaspoon of sea salt and bring the water to a boil.
4. Remove the mixture from the refrigerator. Wash your hands and take the refrigerated batter and roll it into 1" balls, then add them into the boiling water. Do the same with the remaining batter.
5. Reduce the heat and place a lid over the pot and let it simmer for about 20 minutes.
6. In a separate pot, heat the chicken or vegetable stock.
7. When the matzo balls are finished cooking, remove it from the simmering water and place it into the pot with the chicken or vegetable stock.

Silver Dollar Pancakes

Ingredients:

- 1 ½ cups of blanched almond flour
- ¼ tsp of Celtic sea salt
- ¼ tsp of baking soda
- 3 pcs of large eggs
- 1 tbsp of water
- 1 tbsp of vanilla extract
- 2 tbsp of agave nectar

Directions:

1. In a large mixing bowl, combine the eggs, vanilla extract, water, and agave nectar. Whisk the Ingredients: together until properly incorporated.

2. Add in the almond flour, baking soda, and Celtic sea salt. Stir until the Ingredients: form a smooth batter.
3. Prepare a skillet and heat coconut or grape seed oil over medium heat.
4. Use a large tablespoon to scoop the batter on the skillet. Cook the pancakes one at a time.
5. When the batter becomes bubbly, flip the pancakes to cook the other side. Repeat the procedure with the rest of the batter.

Cinnamon Buns

Ingredients:

For the toppings:

- 1 tbsp of ground cinnamon
- 1 tbsp of grape seed oil
- 2 tbsp of agave nectar

For the bun:

- ¼ tsp of Celtic sea salt
- ¼ cup of grape seed oil
- ¼ cup of agave nectar
- 3 pcs of eggs
- 1 cup of blanched almond flour
- 2 tbsp of coconut flour
- ½ tsp of baking soda

- 1 tbsp of vanilla extract

Directions:

1. Make the toppings by combining the agave nectar, ground cinnamon, and grape seed oil. Whisk the Ingredients: together until well mixed. Then, set it aside.
2. In a large mixing bowl, combine the almond flour, baking soda, coconut flour, and salt. Stir the Ingredients: together.
3. Add in the agave nectar, grape seed oil, eggs, and vanilla extract. Whisk the Ingredients: together until it forms a smooth batter.
4. Prepare a muffin tin and line it with muffin cups. Scoop the batter into the muffin cups filling about ¼ of the way. Then, add in the toppings. Do the same with the rest of the batter and toppings.
5. Place the muffin tin inside the oven and bake for 8 to 12 minutes at 350F. Once done

baking, let it cool for two hours. Best enjoyed with cream cheese frosting.

Potatoes With Eggs And Green Beans

Ingredients:

- 1/8 tsp. red pepper, crushed

- 2 garlic cloves

- ½ tsp. salt

- 4 eggs

- Ground pepper

- 2 Tbsp. olive oil

- 1 c. green beans

- 2 lbs. peeled and diced potatoes

- Paprika

Directions:

1. If you use fresh beans, you can cook them in some water in a saucepan so they become crisp tender, which will take around 3

minutes. Drain this out and place under cold water.
2. Next, heat up some oil in a skillet and heat it up before spreading your potatoes out on the skillet in one layer.
3. Make sure to turn these potatoes over a few times and continue cooking for about 20 minutes.
4. After this time, you can stir in the pepper, salt, red pepper, garlic, and green beans.
5. Take your eggs and crack them in a bowl before slowly adding them into the pan with the vegetables.
6. Cover the skillet and let it cook for about 5 minutes so that the whites have time to set. Sprinkle on some paprika and then serve the dish right away.

Breakfast Smoothies

Ingredients:

- 1 c. mixed berries, frozen
- ¼ c. tofu
- 1/2 banana
- ½ c. apple juice

Directions:

1. Bring out your blender and add in the tofu, apple juice, banana, and berries inside.
2. Turn the blender on and let the Ingredients: blend until they become smooth.
3. Pour into your favorite glass and then enjoy.

Blueberry Pancakes

Ingredients:

- 1 egg
- 500 ml. milk
- 150 g. blueberries
- 1 banana
- 15 g. butter
- 1 tsp. baking powder
- 100 g. flour, gluten free

Directions:

1. Place the butter into a bowl and let it melt in the microwave. Once the butter is melted you can whisk it together with the milk and the egg.
2. In another bowl, you can mix the baking powder and the flour. Once they are

combined, stir it in with your milk mixture and continue mixing so that everything is well combined. It is fine if the mixture is a little bit lumpy.

3. Stir the banana and blueberries next before placing the batter into the refrigerator to stand for around 30 minutes.
4. When you are ready, you can heat up some oil on a skillet and spoon some of the batter onto it. Sprinkle the blueberries over the batter.
5. Cook your pancakes for about 3 minutes so that the batter starts to bubble. When that happens, you can turn the pancake over and cook for another 1 ½ minutes.
6. Continue these steps with the rest of the batter before enjoying.

Eggplant And Mango Salad

Ingredients:

- ¼ tsp. ground better
- 2 scallion bunches
- 2 ripe mangoes
- 4 c. romaine lettuce, torn
- ½ a head of broccoli
- ¼ c. chopped cilantro
- ¼ c. chopped peanuts, roasted
- 2 1/3 tsp. chili powder
- 4 Tbsp. olive oil
- 2 ½ tsp. curry powder
- 1/3 c. lemon juice
- 2 eggplants

- ¼ c. salsa
- ¼ tsp. salt
- ¼ c. honey
- 1 ½ c. lentils, cooked

Directions:

1. Start this recipe off by turning on the oven and letting it heat up to 500 degrees.
2. Bring out a bowl and 2 teaspoons of the curry powder and chili powder along with 1 tablespoon of the oil. After this time, you can add the eggplant and broccoli and toss it all well.
3. Spread out this eggplant mixture on a baking sheet and place into the oven to roast for around 15 minutes.
4. Bring out another bowl and combine the pepper, salt, honey, salsa, lemon juice, curry powder, chili powder, and the rest of the oil.

5. When the eggplant is ready, you can add it in along with the scallions and the lentils. Toss everything to combine.
6. Serve this recipe on the romaine lettuce with the cilantro, nuts, and mango before enjoying.

Chocolate Squares

Ingredients:

- Eggs 2
- Vanilla extract 1 teaspoon
- Coconut 2 cups (finely shredded)
- Chocolate chips ½ cup

Directions:

1. Take a small bowl and whisk egg and vanilla together until well combined.
2. Add coconut and chocolate chips and stir well.
3. Pour into the prepared baking pan.
4. Insert into the preheated oven of 180°c and bake for 20 minutes, until top is golden.
5. Cool and cut into squares before serving.

Coconut And Banana Pie

Ingredients:

- Butter 2 tablespoons
- Vanilla extract 1 ½ teaspoons
- Olive oil 2 tablespoons
- Coconut flakes 32 tablespoons (toasted)
- Salt small pinch
- Bananas 4
- Cornstarch ¼ cup
- Sugar 2/3 cup
- Heavy cream 2 cups
- Egg yolks 3

For cream:

- Heavy cream 1 cup

- Vanilla extract ½ teaspoon
- Honey 2 tablespoons (gently melted and cooled)

Directions:

1. Take a medium sized sauce pan and combine the cornstarch, sugar and; whisk cream in gradually. Cook over medium heat, stirring constantly. Whisk until custard is thick, about 2 minutes.
2. In another bowl, beat egg yolks and slowly add some of the hot mass; cook for about couple of minutes, stirring constantly.
3. After removing from the fire, whisk in butter and vanilla to the mixture and set aside.
4. Into the cooled crust place the sliced bananas on the bottom. Pour about half of the mass over the bananas to cover, and top with another layer of the remaining slices and mass; refrigerate until cold.

5. Spread unto chilled pie and top with toasted coconut.

Baby Spinach And Fennel Salad

Ingredients:

- Fennel: 1/2 cup, chopped
- Olive Oil: 1 tablespoon
- Sea Salt: 1/2 teaspoon
- Sunflower seeds: 1/4 cup, shelled
- Turmeric: 1/2 teaspoon
- Almonds: 1/4 cup, slivers
- Apple Cider Vinegar: 1/4 cup.
- Baby spinach: 4 cups
- Cherry Tomatoes: 8, cut in half

Directions:

1. Add Spinach, fennel, sunflower seeds, tomatoes, and almonds in a large bowl.

2. Stir together olive oil, vinegar, salt, and turmeric in a small bowl.
3. Pour vinaigrette over salad and toss well.

Bacon Bleu Cheese Burger Patties

Ingredients:

- Egg: 1 large

- Ground Beef: 1 pound

- Red Onion: 1/4 cup, finely chopped

- Sea Salt: 1/2 teaspoon

- Almond Meal: 1/4 cup

- Bacon: 4 strips, cut into 1/4 inch pieces

- Black Pepper: 1/2 teaspoon

- Bleu Cheese Crumbles: 1/2 cup

Directions:

1. Cook bacon pieces in a skillet over medium heat, stirring frequently, until crisp, about 5 minutes. Remove bacon from pan, retain bacon grease.

2. Combine Ground beef, egg, almond meal, salt, pepper, onion, bleu cheese crumbles and cooked bacon in a large bowl, mix well by hand.
3. Divide meat mixture into fourths, and form into patties.
4. Cook in skillet containing bacon grease over medium heat, flipping once during cooking until ground beef is cooked through, about 5 minutes per side.

Bacon Lettuce Tomato Salad

Ingredients:

- 1 handful cilantro, minced
- 1 handful feta cheese
- 1 tsp. mustard
- Juice from a lemon
- 3 ounces olive oil
- 1 ½ ounces balsamic vinegar
- Lettuce, chopped in bitesized pieces
- 4 slices bacon, cooked and crumbled
- ½ cucumber, diced
- 1 avocado, diced
- 2 handfuls cherry tomatoes, diced

- Sea salt

Directions:

1. Place the lettuce, cucumber, cilantro, avocado and cherry tomatoes in a large bowl.
2. Add the cooked and chopped bacon, followed by the feta cheese. Mix the Ingredients: together and transfer into a serving bowl.
3. In a small bowl, mix the olive oil, vinegar, lemon juice and mustard together. Add a sprinkle of sea salt and stir. This is the dressing.
4. Drizzle the dressing over the salad and toss to coat.

Cheddar Broccoli Soup

Ingredients:

- 2 carrots, diced
- 1 yellow onion, diced

- 10 ounces broccoli florets

- 2 cups cheddar cheese, shredded

- Sea salt, to taste

- 1 Tbsp. butter, unsalted

- ½ + ¼ tsp. sea salt

- 2 ½ cups vegetable stock

- Ground black pepper, to taste

Directions:

1. Heat the butter in a large pot. Stir in ¼ tsp. of sea salt and the diced onions. Sauté for about 8 minutes.
2. Add the carrots and the broccoli florets and stir. Pour just enough vegetable stock into the pot so that it covers the vegetables.
3. Turn the heat on the stove up to high and bring the vegetable stock to a boil.

4. Turn the heat down and cover the pot. Let the mixture simmer for about 10 minutes. The broccoli and the carrots should be tender. If not, let them simmer for a little bit longer.
5. Remove the pot from the heat and add the remaining ½ tsp. of sea salt and stir. Sprinkle the cheddar cheese into the mixture and stir until smooth. If necessary, add more vegetable stock.
6. Allow the mixture to cool. Once cool, pour a little of the mixture into a food processor and blend until smooth. Continue in this manner until you have blended all the mixture. Add the smoothed mixture back into the pot. If you find it is too thick, add a bit more vegetable stock until you achieve the desired consistency.
7. Place the pot back on the stove and warm. Season with salt and pepper to taste. Serve while warm.

Bbq Meat Loaf

Ingredients:

- ¼ cup grated reducedfat Parmesan cheese
- ¼ cup lowfat sour cream
- 2 garlic cloves, minced
- ½ cup diced red bell peppers,
- 1 cup BBQ Sauce
- 2 pounds 7% fat ground beef
- 2 egg whites
- 2 Weetabix biscuits, crushed
- Salt and pepper

Directions:

1. Preheat oven to 350 degrees F.
2. Mix all Ingredients: in a large bowl.

3. Form the mixture into two loaves.
4. Set shallow rack on a jelly roll pan and place loaves on top of the rack. Bake on center shelf for 1 hour.
5. Remove from oven, top with BBQ sauce, and bake until the sauce becomes thick and dark, about 20 minutes more.

Chicken With Basil Cream Sauce

Ingredients:

- 2 medium red onions, cut into ¼inch wide strips
- 2 cups loosely packed basil
- 2 teaspoons Watkins™ or Molly McButter®
- 5 cloves minced garlic
- ¼ cup fatfree chicken broth
- 4 teaspoons olive oil (2 teaspoons + 2 teaspoons)
- 6 (4ounce) skinless chicken breasts
- 16 ounces lowfat cottage cheese
- 4 ½ teaspoons ZSweet®
- 4 bell peppers (one each: red, green, yellow, and orange), cut into ¼inch wide strips

- Salt and pepper

Directions:

1. To make the sauce, place cottage cheese, butter flavoring, Sweat®, basil, and chicken broth in the work bowl of a food processor. Blend until smooth. Season with salt and pepper to taste.
2. Heat 2 teaspoons of olive oil in a large skillet over medium high heat. Season chicken breasts with salt and pepper. Cook until well browned, about 6 8 minutes on each side. Transfer chicken to a plate and cover with aluminum foil.
3. Heat the remaining 2 teaspoons of olive oil over medium high heat. Add peppers and onions to skillet. Season with salt and pepper. Cook and stir until tender, about 6 minutes.
4. Stir in the garlic and heat until fragrant, about 30 seconds.

5. Cut the chicken across the grain at a slight angle into thin strips.
6. Combine chicken and sauce with the vegetables. Cook and stir for 2 minutes.

bq Potatoes

Ingredients:

- 2 tablespoons paprika
- 2 tablespoons Sweat
- 2 teaspoons salt
- 1 teaspoon ground chipotle pepper
- ½ teaspoon pepper
- ½ teaspoon garlic powder
- 4 pounds Yukon gold potatoes, about 10 potatoes
- 1 tablespoon olive oil
- ½ teaspoon onion powder

Directions:

1. Preheat oven to 450 degrees F.

2. Cut potatoes in wedges by first cutting each in half along the longest edge and then cutting each half into three wedges.
3. Mix paprika, Sweat, salt, chipotle, pepper, garlic, and onion in a small bowl.
4. In a large bowl, toss potatoes with olive oil.
5. Sprinkle potatoes with half of the spice mixture and toss.
6. Sprinkle potatoes with the remaining spice mixture and toss.
7. Arrange each potato wedge on a jelly roll pan with one of the cut edges facing down.
8. Cover pan with aluminum foil and bake on the middle oven shelf for 20 minutes.
9. Remove aluminum foil and bake potatoes until golden brown, about 30 40 minutes more.

Strawberry Banana Smoothie

Ingredients:

- 1 can coconut milk
- ½ cup ice cubes
- 1 cup fresh strawberries
- 1 fresh banana

Directions:

1. Cut strawberries and banana into pieces, put all the Ingredients: in a Blender or Vitamix and blend until smooth.
2. Enjoy chilled

Crusted Chicken Tenders

Ingredients:

- 6 chicken tenders
- 1 cups vegetable oil
- 1 tbsp. honey
- 1 tbsp. mustard
- 1 packet corn tortillas
- ½ cup almond flour
- ½ cup buttermilk

Directions:

1. Crush the tortillas to crumb like consistency. Keep in a large bowl.
2. In a medium bowl, keep almond flour and in another buttermilk. Drench chicken in buttermilk first, then in flour, shaking off

excess. Then dip in tortilla crumbs. Transfer to large plate or baking sheet.

3. In large skillet, heat oil over medium heat. Cook chicken well to crusty about 12 minutes. Transfer to paper towels.//
4. In a small bowl, mix the mustard and honey. Serve chicken with sauce.

Glazed Salmon

Ingredients:

- A pinch of garlic salt
- A pinch of pepper
- 1 lb salmon
- ¼ cup maple syrup
- 4 tsp soy sauce
- 1 clove garlic, minced

Directions:

1. Preheat your oven to 400F.
2. Place the salmon on a baking dish and glaze it with the maple dressing previously made.
3. Bake for 20 minutes, or until the salmon disintegrates upon light pressure.

Vegetable Chili

Ingredients:

- 2*4oz canned green chilli peppers, drained
- ¼ cup chilli powder
- 1 tsp ground cumin
- 2 tbsp dried oregano
- 1 tbsp ground black pepper
- 1*14oz canned kidney beans, drained
- 2*12 oz vegetarian burger crumbles
- 3 tsp olive oil
- ½ medium onion, chopped
- 2 bay leaves
- 3 green bell peppers, chopped
- 2 jalapeno peppers, chopped

- 1 tbsp salt
- 1 stalks celery, chopped
- 3 cloves garlic, chopped
- 6*14oz canned chopped tomatoes
- 1*14oz canned garbanzo beans, drained
- 1*14oz canned black beans

Directions:

1. In a large saucepan, warm 3 tbsp of olive oil over a high heat. Toss in the onion, garlic and bay leaves, oregano, cumin and a pinch of salt.
2. Cook for 57 minutes or until the onions have softened. Next, add celery, green bell peppers , jalapeno peppers & green chilli peppers.
3. Cook for 1015 minutes or until all the vegetables have softened. Stir continuously throughout to ensure nothing burns.

4. Next, add the vegetable burger protein. Lower the temperature until there is a mild simmer. Cover and leave to simmer gently for 57 minutes.
5. After this, add the chopped tomatoes to the saucepan, alongside the chilli powder, pepper and beans.
6. Raise the heat and bring the content of the pan to a boil. Cover, reduce the heat and cook for 45 minutes.
7. Remove the lid and add the corn. Cook for 5 more minutes. Finally serve immediately.

Berry Coconut Smoothie

Ingredients:

- ½ cup plain yogurt
- ½ cup vanilla or unflavored whey protein powder
- 1 tablespoon ground flaxseeds
- ¼ cup blackberries, blueberries, strawberries, or any kind of berries
- ½ cup coconut milk
- ½ teaspoon coconut extract
- 4 ice cubes

Directions:

1. Mix the yogurt, coconut milk, whey protein, berries, coconut extract, flaxseed, and ice

cubes together. Mix until the texture turns smooth. Serve immediately.

Ginger Blueberry Parfait

Ingredients:

- 1 cup part skim ricotta cheese
- 1 tablespoon grated peeled fresh ginger
- 4 tablespoons maple syrup
- 1 cup blueberries
- 1 peeled, chopped, and pitted avocado
- 4 sprigs fresh mint

Directions:

1. Mix the ginger, blueberries, and 1 tablespoon of maple syrup in a bowl. Leave it for about 5 minutes.
2. Mix the ricotta, avocado, and 3 tablespoons maple syrup inside the processor.
3. Pound the mixture. Then lay on the ricotta mixture and the blueberry mixture on dessert

dishes or in 4 parfait glasses, and top with berries and mint leaves and serve.

Flourless Honey Almond Cake

Ingredients:

- 1½ cups toasted whole almonds
- 1 teaspoon vanilla extract
- 4 large eggs
- ½ cup honey
- ½ teaspoon baking soda
- ½ teaspoon salt

Topping

- ¼ cup toasted sliced almonds
- 2 tablespoons honey

Directions:

1. Preheat oven to 175°C. Cover the pan with cooking spray. Put on the parchment paper and spray the paper at the bottom.
2. Place the whole almonds in a blender or food processor until they are finely ground. Add 4 egg yolks, ½cup honey, baking soda, vanilla, and sea salt in a bowl, mix well. Put in the ground almonds and continue mixing
3. Put 4 egg whites in another bowl with the electric until it becomes foamy and doubled in volume. With a spatula, put in the egg whites into the nut mixture until they're mixed well.
4. Bake for about 28 minutes and it turns golden brown. Leave it for 10 minutes to cool down. Remove by running a knife around the pan's edges and remove the side ring gently.

Oriental Chicken Salad

Ingredients:

- ¼ cup sliced almonds
- ½ teaspoon wasabi powder
- 1 teaspoon ground ginger
- 4 chicken breasts without bone, sliced and skinless
- 4 cups mixed greens
- 2 large eggs
- ½ cup of finely ground golden flaxseeds
- 2 tablespoons coconut flour
- 1 tablespoon onion powder
- ½ cup of Asian dipping sauce

Directions:

1. Preheat the oven to 400 degrees Fahrenheit
2. Whisk the eggs in a shallow bowl
3. In another shallow bowl combine the flaxseeds, coconut flour onion powder wasabi powder and ginger and mix
4. Dip each chicken strip in the eggs and then roll in the flaxseed mixture
5. Place each strip on a baking sheet
6. Bake for 20minutes turning once
7. Divide the greens among 4 plates
8. Sprinkle the almonds and drizzle with vinaigrette
9. Top with chicken strips

Chicken Nuggets

Ingredients:

- ¼ teaspoon garlic powder

- ¼ teaspoon sea salt

- ½ cup parmesan cheese, grated

- ¼ teaspoon ground black pepper
- 1 pound of chicken breasts, without bone or skin
- 2 eggs
- 2 tablespoons of melted butter
- ¼ teaspoon onion powder
- ½ cup of ground flaxseeds

Directions:

1. Preheat the oven to 375oF
2. Use parchment paper to line a rimmed baking sheet
3. Slice the chicken into 1½inch pieces
4. Whisk the eggs and butter
5. Mix the flaxseeds, onion powder, cheese, salt, garlic powder and pepper in another separate bowl

6. Coat each chicken piece with the egg mixture and then the flaxseed mixture
7. Place the chicken on a baking pan
8. Bake for 20minutes turning once

Dreamy Walnut Cake

Ingredients:

- 2 ounces butter

- ¼ teaspoon salt

- 4 egg whites

- 4 egg yolks

- ½ cup dark walnuts

- 1 ½ cups English walnuts

- 1 cup sugar (separated into segments of two ¼ cups and ½ cup)

Directions:

1. Toast the pecans first, and afterward let them cool. Grind them finely along with ¼ cup of sugar.

2. In a little pot, cream the spread in addition to a half cup of sugar. The combination needs to become feathery and light.
3. Add the yolks into the blend each in turn. Scratch the bowl, particularly the sides, and afterward beat subsequent to adding one yolk.
4. Fold in the pecans into the egg and margarine combination. Set aside.
5. In an oil free bowl, whisk the egg whites and gradually include the last ¼ cup of sugar. You will see the arrangement of solid pinnacles.
6. Delicately overlay in this blend into the spread combination. Overlay in just a little at a time until everything has been completely and equitably mixed.
7. Pour the substance into a little Bundt or portion pan.

www.ingramcontent.com/pod-product-compliance
Lightning Source LLC
LaVergne TN
LVHW010224070526
838199LV00062B/4723